Rabea Koshak

Early Return To Work Program In Saudi Arabia

Rabea Koshak

Early Return To Work Program In Saudi Arabia

Implementation, for Employees with Low Back Pain

LAP LAMBERT Academic Publishing

Imprint

Any brand names and product names mentioned in this book are subject to trademark, brand or patent protection and are trademarks or registered trademarks of their respective holders. The use of brand names, product names, common names, trade names, product descriptions etc. even without a particular marking in this work is in no way to be construed to mean that such names may be regarded as unrestricted in respect of trademark and brand protection legislation and could thus be used by anyone.

Cover image: www.ingimage.com

Publisher:
LAP LAMBERT Academic Publishing
is a trademark of
International Book Market Service Ltd., member of OmniScriptum Publishing Group
17 Meldrum Street, Beau Bassin 71504, Mauritius

ISBN: 978-3-659-49301-0

Copyright © Rabea Koshak
Copyright © 2013 International Book Market Service Ltd., member of OmniScriptum Publishing Group

Content

Acknowledgment	3
1. Introduction	4
1.1 Background	4
1.2. Description of the problem	4
1.3. Outline of the work	4
2. Literature review	6
2.1 Conditions associated with low back pain	7
2.2 Pain and Disability	9
2.3. Impairment and Disability	9
2.4 Effectiveness of early returns to work	10
2.5. General description of the early return to work program	12
2.6. Problem statement and study questions	15
3. Methodology	17
3.1. Study design	17
3.2. Employees	17
3.2.1. Development of the questionnaire & measurement instruments	17
3.2.2. Selection of respondents	17
3.3. Employers	19
3.3.1 Development of interview	19
3.3.2. Selection of the respondents	20
3.4. Social Insurance organization	21
3.4.1. Development of interview	22
3.4.2. Selection of the respondents	22
3.5. Data analysis	23
4. Results	24
4.1. Employees	24
4.1.1. Characteristics of the respondents	24
4.1.2. Employees attitude towards low back pain and ERTW programs	25
4.1.3. Willingness of the employees to participate in ERTW programs	27
4.2. Employers	29
4.2.1. Problem of Sickness absenteeism due to low back pain and RTW policy	29
4.2.2. Positively about development of early return to work program	30
4.2.3. Willingness to implement ERTW program	30
4.3. Social Insurance organization	32
4.3.1. Cost problem of low back pain	32
4.3.2. Positive attitude towards development of ERTW program	33
4.3.3. Willingness to support the implementation ERTW program	33

4.3.4. Possibility to participate in ERTW program for employees and employers	34
5. Conclusion, Discussion and Recommendations	36
5.1. Limitations	36
5.2. Conclusion	36
5.3. Discussion	38
5.4. Recommandations	39
Appendixes	
A. Employees' questionnaire	42
B. Check-list interview with employers	45
C. Check-list interview with social insurance policy makers	46
References	47

ACKNOWLEDGMENT

At this moment after an intensive work, I look back upon a great experience and the product of my attempt to learn about work and health and early reintegration of disabled people.

This work consist of results collected from the questionnaire and interviews of the three group of this study, the employees, employers and social insurance organization policy makers in Saudi Arabia.

The text brings together visions regarding the implementation of early return to work program in Saudi Arabia. This would have never been successful without those who were involved in the preparation and arrangement of the conducted interviews and who give a hand in the distribution of the questionnaires.

I also owe special thanks for my wife and my two boys who supported me and shared with me my intensive work.

Rabea Koshak, July 2009

1. Introduction

1.1. Background

Musculoskeletal diseases (MSD) are one of the most common causes of sickness, absence, long term incapability of work and health retirement. Needless to say, persistent low back pain is a major health and socio-economic problem and so, preventing workplace injuries and illness is the responsibility of everyone at the workplace (OSHA, 2009). Whenever an injury or illness occurs, it is important for both the employer as well as the incapacitated worker to minimize the human and financial impact, by getting the worker back to a safe and productive working environment as soon as medically possible (Waddell, 2004).

It has been shown recently, that rest and the avoidance of action do not help in the recovery of people with low back pain. Taking too much rest may lead to a prolonged recovery time and probably chronic back pain. Therefore, it appears to be much better to keep a normal level of day-to-day activity to help in the recovery process and returning to work and regular life activities (Wheeler, 1995).

Usual treatments have failed to reduce the load of chronic low back pain (LBP), and physicians not following guidelines may have contributed to this problem (Waddell, 1987). Therefore, early return to work programs was developed in search for new solutions (Mayer, 1985). The initial ideas of an early return to work programs for patients with disabling chronic low back pain were projected by Mayer et al. (Mayer, 1985).

1.2. Description of the problem

Despite the development of health services and facilities in Saudi Arabia and the government attention for the Saudi health sector and to enhance the well-being of citizens in the Kingdom, still no reintegration programs exists. In Saudi Arabia, low back pain is an important problem that leads to a high level of medical and social costs. Therefore, it will be important to look for possibilities to develop programs for employees with low back pain in Saudi Arabia. In this work, we will study the feasibility of implementing early reintegration in Saudi Arabian organizations.

1.3. Outline of the work

In the following chapter, we will give a literature review on low back pain and early return to work (ERTW) issues in addition to the problem statement and the study questions. In chapter three, we are going to explain the methods we used in this work to get to chapter four, that will lay out the results. Chapter five gives the limitations, conclusion, discussion, and the recommendations to this work.

2. Literature review

In this chapter, we will shed some light on the Disability Management (DM) policy and its importance in the organizations in applying an ERTW program. We will also mention the common causes of low back pain (2.1.). The whole idea of this work is to study the implementation of ERTW program and how it decrease the disability, therefore it would be important to give differences between a disability with low back pain (2.2.) and a disability resulting from an impairment (2.3.) because each disability has its own rules and dealing with one differs than the other. Sections (2.4.) and (2.5.) of this chapter are going to give us a general idea on both, the effectiveness of ERTW program and how such a program works. Last section (2.6.) will display problem statement and study questions of this book.

The problems associated with Disability Management are complex by nature; therefore, we face a lot of difficulties in developing Disability Management strategies. First a need assessment has to be performed to gain information about work disruption problems and their related consequences. The second step would be the definition of goal and objectives. Depending on the organization's emphasizes there are several different inferior aims. When goals and objectives are established, Disability Management strategies can be developed to intervene on work disruption problems. (Millington & Strauser, 1998).

Today, disability managements' main target is directed towards achieving a lower absence rate, keeping healthy and productive employees, increasing the participation of people with disabilities and reintegration programs improvement (Whitaker, 2001). There are many principles of disability management that includes interdisciplinary team, proactive intervention and early intervention. Proactive team can involve many different expertises ranging from physician, psychologists, and occupational therapists to human resources manager and risk managers. They work together as a treatment team in sorting out work disrupting problems and in the planning, implementation and evaluation of disability management. Not only are Proactive interventions responsible for accident prevention and safety programs (Shrey & Hursh, 1999). But, they also focus at workers 'at risk' behavior such as drug and alcohol abuse, stress in workplace etc. (Millington & Strauser, 1998; Shrey & Hursh, 1999). Smoking cessation clinics, stress management programs and corporate fitness centers are all examples of such interventions (Shrey & Hursh, 1999, Bratton & Gold, 2007).

Disability management has an important principle which is the early intervention which has attained broad acceptance among various disability benefits system, especially workers compensation and long term disability insurance carriers.

By early returning to work employees can maintain their occupational bonding with their organization, this in turn will motivate them toward faster recovery, and helps them gaining insights in cultural barriers and adjustment possibilities of organizations (Millington & Strauser, 1998).

Early return to work interventions should emphasize the facilitation of monitoring and coordination. Monitoring necessitates that disabled employees should receive information about their medical treatment, and fill them with possible jobsite accommodations and other resources in the return-to-work process, that's why it should be an effective coordination and a continuous contact between the disabled employee, employers, treatment team, case management, etc.(Shrey & Hursh, 1999).

2.1. Conditions associated with low back pain

Low back pain is a prevalent, clinically complex phenomenon. Many factors increase the risk of developing low back pain. Some of these factors are considered important risk factors for the development of persistent low back pain. As people age, bone strength, muscle elasticity and tone tend to decrease. The discs of the vertebral column begin to lose their fluid and flexibility, which decreases their ability to cushion the vertebrae.

Pain can occur when, for example, someone lifts something that is too heavy or when one overstretches, causing a sprain, strain, or spasm in one of the muscles or ligaments in the back. If the spine becomes overly strained or compressed, a disc may rupture or bulge outward. This rupture may put pressure on one of the more than 50 nerves rooted to the spinal cord that controls the body movements and transmit signals from the body to the brain. In other words, nerve roots compression or irritation results in back pain (Devereaux 2009).

Low back pain can be caused by a wide variety of factors. These include structural problems of the back, inflammation, infections, muscle and soft tissue injury, secondary response to other diseases or conditions, imbalances in body mechanics, life style causing obesity, and weight gain during pregnancy, smoking, stress, poor physical condition, and psychological/social factors, among others. Additionally, scar tissue created when the injured back heals itself does not have the strength or flexibility of normal tissue. Buildup of scar tissue from repeated injuries eventually weakens the back and can lead to more serious injury (Waddell, 2004).

There are many conditions that may cause low back pain and requires treatment by a physician or other health specialist (Devereaux 2009). However, a substantial proportion of patients who develop chronic low back pain have no identifiable structural pathology capable of explaining the pain. Pain specialists sometimes attribute the pain in these patients to unknown musculoskeletal factors; sometimes the term "idiopathic" is used and means that the cause is entirely unknown.

Occasionally, a more serious medical problem related to low back pain may arise when the pain is accompanied by fever or loss of bowel or bladder control; a pain when coughing, and progressive weakness in the legs may indicate a pinched nerve or other serious condition.

Another important aspect for causing the pain that is not to be taken lightly is the psychological side and how the psychological as well as the social factors can tremendously increase the risk of low back pain. Various studies show that psychological factors can be a cause in the development of low back pain. These factors include anxiety, depression, somatization symptoms, traumatic responsibility, job dissatisfaction, mental fatigue at work, and negative beliefs. In one study, various symptoms causing psychological distress played a role in the development of back disorders in people who did not have previous back pain (Nachemson, A., 1999). In one study, low job satisfaction showed to be a risk factors for sickness absence due to low back pain. Other studies showed a relation between low social support (from supervisors or co-workers) and sickness absence due to low back pain (Hoogendoorn, W.E., et al 2002).

People who control their pain or have strategies to cope with pain are in fact lucky, as they can adjust their life to their pain as one research noted (Simmonds, 1996). Some researchers have the belief that psychological factors as previously mentioned are considered primary causes of low back pain (Sarno, 1991). A secondary cause is distress regardless of being the result of pain or physical restriction, may aggravate pain and therefore disability (Simmonds 1996). When pain causes stress or stress causes pain, a vicious cycle is established, and in either ways both will produce more stress, which again can causes more low back strain and pain.

The quality of life of the individual and his/ her family will be affected once low back pain has occurred. This will often have a disruptive influence and will produce an advantage for the patient in ways of increasing the family's attention or support toward the patient. Keeping in mind these kinds of reactions to chronic pain is an important part of having a successful treatment (Stenger, 1992).

2.2. Back pain and Disability

Back pain and disability may appear to be having the same meaning. They are obviously related but we must make a very clear conceptual distinction between them as they are not the same.

Pain is a symptom, in other words, it's not diagnosis, a disease or even a clinical sign. (Merskey 1979) give the best definition of pain: "An unpleasant sensory and emotional experience associated with actual or potential tissue damage, or described in terms of such damage"

Pain cannot be assessed directly so we need to depend on the patients' experience, how he or she thinks and feel and how he or she communicates with it.

Disability is a restricted activity. The standard definition is by the World Health Organization (WHO): "Any restriction or lack of ability to perform an activity in the manner or within the range considered normal for a human being".

Assessment of disability is again a subjective matter, i.e.: it depends on the patient's own reports of what they can and cannot do.

Failure to distinguish between pain and disability has a major impact on management. Many doctors, therapists and patients assume or believe that the disability is caused by the pain and by treating the pain, the disability will disappear. Pain and disability are clearly related to each other, but have different aspects on illness as mentioned earlier. For example: having back pain does not always lead to disability and furthermore, the amount of disability is not always proportionate to the severity of pain. We often see patients who manage to lead a normal life despite the severe pain, while other patients are totally or permanently disabled while having mild pain.

2.3. Impairment and Disability

The American Medical Association (AMA) has pointed out clearly the differences between impairment and disability. Impairment has as a medical perception, as it is a consequence of a disease or an illness that leads to a change in one's health status. Disability however, is a vocational concept. In real life situations, a particular impairment depending on particular work conditions can have a different amount of disability. For example, a total amputation of a musicians' single finger can put him/ her out of work. However, the same amputation of the same finger will have no harm on a truck driver. That is to say: same impairment, different disability (Walker 1993).

Accepting the distinction between impairment and a disability has liberated many companies in the United States of America. Hence, the risk management and Human resource (HR) personnel can now reintegrate the impaired employees back to work by modifying the work settings to the worker's impairments in order to fit the workers limitations. Thus, really reducing or eliminating any disability. Therefore, disability is in fact manageable. Particularly if both employer and employee are fine with the work modifications, in that case disability management can be a win-win human resource outcome (Walker 1993).

2.4. Effectiveness of early return to work programs

This section provides an overview of empirical evidence for ERTW programs. The outcome of the early return to work program was found to have a significant improvement on the psychological status, perceived pain, disability and work capability based on a study report that was sustained for 24 months in the United Kingdom (Hunter 2006).

During the recovery period, some work activities may or can still be performed by most injured workers and by doing so, they return to daily work and life activities sooner than they would have and this actually help in the recovery process (Koopman, 2004).

In fact, the longer a worker is off work due to injury or illness, the lower the likelihood that they will return to work if ever. It is a high priority to help patients to return to work as soon as medically possible since it's clearly beneficial for both the employer and injured. In other words, the injured worker will benefit by staying productively active, needless to say accelerating healing/ recovery process as well as restoring their source of income.

Hildebrandt (1997), Frank et al (1998) and Molde (2004), clarify different advantages of early return to work for the employees, employers and social insurance organization:

- Avoidance of wage loss: Workers' Compensation benefits replace only part of the employee's wages. Therefore, the earlier an employee returns to work, the faster their income will return to its pre-injury level.
- Faster recuperation: Current medical guidance dictates that Soft-tissue injures will require only a little rest in order to avoid destructive muscles atrophy. This comes in response to workers' Compensation claims
- Positive social reintegration: As not to feel forgotten by their co-workers by being away from work for long periods due to injuries.

- Avoidance of "disability syndrome": This is a vicious cycle; the longer the employee stays out of the workplace, the more they see themselves as disabled and this makes it more difficult to re-establish the more rigorous discipline of being in the workplace eight hours a day (Hansen, 2005).
- Improved self-worth: The feeling of self satisfaction or sense of contribution to our own skills and abilities that most if not all of us feel will be lost if an employee stays off work for longer periods.

These were some of the employees' benefits; it would be worthwhile to put some highlight on the employer benefit from early returns to work as well:

- Employers retain valuable workers, restore labor force participation and reduce the negative financial impacts of disability.
- Less funding would be spent on claims due to reduced claims duration
- The need to pay more overtimes to get work normally performed by workers who are absent will be tremendously reduced.
- The effort of recruiting and training of new employees to replace injured/ill workers will be reduced not to mention the costs of the whole process.
- There will be minimum lost productivity due to early returning of experienced workers back to work.
- Fewer employees ending up as long-term disability.

Many social security systems have a major concern in terms of having a high level of expenditure on sickness and disability benefits and decreasing labor participation. Hence, social security systems may in fact benefit from the early return to work program also for instance as follows:

- A quick recovery of injured worker's is in order with returning to work and thus the financial impact of a workers' compensation will be reduced.
- Reductions in both compensation claims due to low back pain as well as ill health retirements, this economic benefit was updated and proved by the study Karrholm, (2008).
- Governments retain tax payers whose reliance on the social safety net is reduced
- Post-treatment work restrictions and sickness absence will be reduced.

2.5. General description of an early return to work program

An early return to work program is generally based on a cost-effective protocol for employees with low back pain (Loisel 1997). Participatory ergonomics is the basis on which the protocol is based on (de Jong, 2002), and it is applied as a means of tertiary prevention.

All around the glob an early return to work program is a systematic approach that needs to begin by a consultation with the occupational physician (Figure1). Accomplishing an agreement about return to work (RTW) plan is the aim of the workplace intervention, and this is done by having active participation and a strong obligation from both the employee and his/ her employer; this needs to be supervised by an RTW coordinator.

The job of an RTW coordinator is to give guidelines of the process in order to reach harmony between both the employee and the employer about an RTW plan. It is essential to have a dynamic participation of both employees and employer in order to attain a concrete basis to implement an RTW plan (Poiraudeau, 2007).

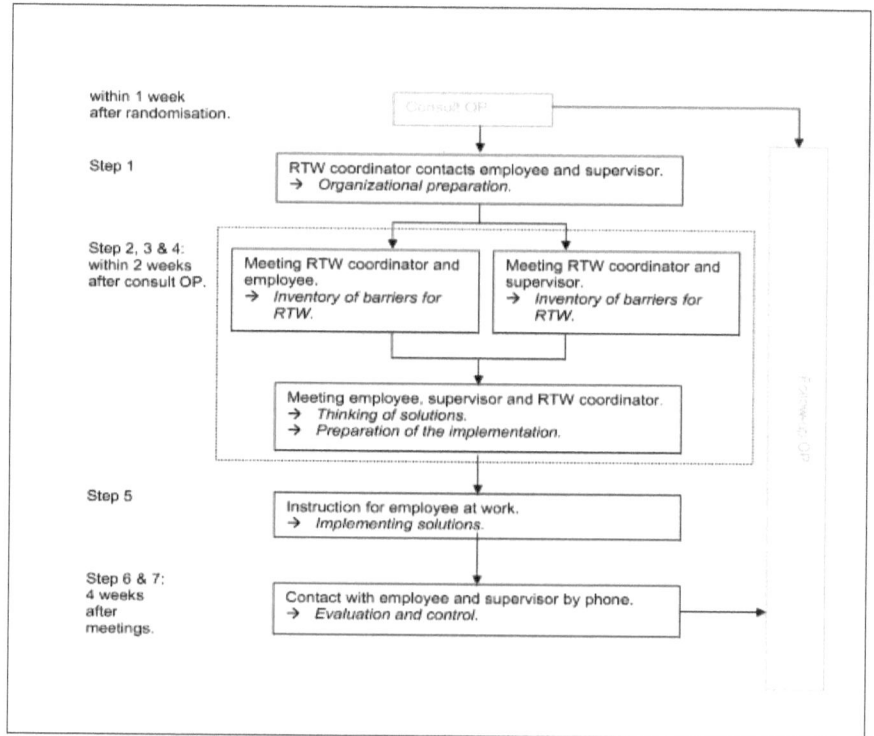

Figure 1: General content of ERTW program (Van Oostrom, 2007)

Occupational Physician Consultation (OP)

Before starting the first step in an intervention plan, all employees must consult an occupational physician. The consultation must take its usual protocol steps (the usual care). The occupational physician will have the employees participate in homework assignment to find out the inventory for stressors, and extra consults may be in order to control or reduce stress even before the intervention starts. Another responsibility of the occupational physician is to enlighten the employer about the workplace intervention and to ask for their participation. To avoid any conflicting advice about RTW the OP sends out a letter to the employee's treating physician regarding the workplace intervention. Like in usual care, it is a necessity for the occupational physician to give an estimate or advice about the date of work re-commencement.

Organizational preparation

The RTW coordinator sits down with the employer and discuss the matter regarding the intervention plan until they agrees about it. Next step would be to inform the person who is responsible for work adjustments and procedures that are to be followed; The RTW coordinator is the one to decide the person in charge.
A meeting is arranged between the employee, employer and the RTW coordinator, along with a checklist with questions about barriers for RTW (Anema, 2003). During these meetings the RTW coordinator will emphasize that the plan of RTW does not necessitate the urgency or the immediate return of the employee.

Inventory of barriers for RTW

The meeting between the RTW coordinator and the employee begins with a visit to the work place, to monitor the employee's workplace. There will be a discussion about the elements of work atmosphere, the teamwork, work satisfaction and work organization. This will give a complete broader picture of the work situation to the RTW coordinator.

The employee is then interviewed by the RTW coordinator; this is to acquire a full description of the main tasks and precise features of these tasks. Barriers are pointed out for each task. However, the barriers are judged on the bases of frequency and severity of these barriers.

A meeting is subsequently arranged between the RTW coordinator and the employer to select the barriers for RTW of the employee from the employers' point of view, and vice a versa is going to happen in the interview between the RTW coordinator and the employee. The RTW coordinator then, makes a summary about the results of the two interviews and comes out with the barriers that are going to be discussed in the next upcoming meeting.

Thinking of solutions

After separate meetings with the employee and then with the employer, another meeting is in order with the employee, the employer and the RTW coordinator to come up together with an outline or solutions for implementation these solutions. When an agreement takes place, the barriers are solved. It is then that the RTW coordinator explains the procedure. Accordingly, the technique (Anema, 2003) and plan they think of will be a collection of ideas from each solution. Prior to being prioritized, all ideas must be judged based on criteria of feasibility, availability, and solving capability of the solution. The main goal is to reach an agreement between the employee and employer in regard to the most feasible solutions.

Preparation of the implementation

The employee, the employer and the RTW coordinator, sits together and try to formulate a plan for implementation of the solutions. This plan describes how this is designed to occur, when the solution is to be implemented, and who is responsible for the implementation of a solution (Anema 2007). A statement about this plan for implementation of solutions must be written by the RTW coordinator and a copy of it is sent to the employee, the employer and the occupational physician.

Implementation of solutions

In the weeks following the meetings, the solutions are implemented. An RTW coordinator will meet with the employee to instruct and give advice to the employee in the workplace. Dealing with new equipment or performing a new job is a good example. The employer can also be educated at the same time, about ways to encourage and guide his employee in their new adjusted work situation.

Evaluation by the RTW coordinator and follow-up by the Occupational Physician

In one month time after the meeting, the employee as well as the employer is contacted by the RTW coordinator to see whether or not the solutions that have been implemented have worked successfully and whether it has contributed to RTW program.

Finally, the RTW coordinator sends out a final report, which unfolds the progression and the results of the implementation and assigns additional guidance to the occupational physician.

2.6. Problem statement and study questions

Low back pain is an important topic in Saudi Arabia; it brings a lot of costs medically, socially and financially. Therefore, it will be important to look for possibilities to develop a program for employees with low back pain in Saudi Arabia (Al-Arfaj, 2003).

The problem of the study can be stated in the following question: "How feasible will it be to implement early return to work programs for employees with low back pain in Saudi Arabian organizations?" From this problem statement, we developed a number of questions to work with.

In the line with the advantages of the early return to work program described above, there are different target groups that can be identified, the most important players in this field are: employees, employers and the social insurance organization, therefore in our study we will consider these different target groups.

To answer the problem statement we will consider the position and opinions of three different actors: employees, employers and social insurance, regarding the following questions:

Employees:
1. Do employees with low back pain have a positive attitude towards early return to work programs?
2. Are employees with low back pain willing to participate in such a program?

Employers:
3. Is there a problem in organizations related to low back pain in Saudi Arabia?
4. Do employers have a positive attitude towards development of early return to work programs?
5. Are the employers willing to implement such a program in their own organizations?

Social insurance organization:
- 6- Is the cost of the low back pain a problem for the social insurance organization?
- 7- Do social insurance policy makers think that early return to work programs could be cost saving?
- 8- Are social insurance policy makers willing to support the implementation of such a program?
- 9- Do social insurance policy makers think that the employees and employers will support such a program?

3. Methodology

In order to answer the question of the feasibility of implementation of early return to work program in Saudi Arabia, it is necessary to do the study on three different perspectives the employees, employers and the social insurance organization policy makers.

3.1. Study design

In this study we will send out a survey to 50 employees, and we will carry out interviews with four employers, one Human Resource consultant and with two representatives of the social insurance organization policy makers. Hence, this study adopted a mixture of method approached: we collected and analyzed both quantitative and qualitative data.

Based on the result of these three groups it can be estimated whether the implementation of early return to work program for employees with low back pain would be successful in Saudi Arabia.

3.2. Employees

Study questions:
1. Do employees with low back pain have a positive attitude towards early return to work programs?
2. Are employees with low back pain willing to participate in such a program?

3.2.1. Development of the questionnaire and measurement instruments

The layout of the questionnaire has been changed several times as we tried to take into account the perspective of the employees regarding the early return to work program in different topics and from different perspectives, until we reached the final step as is shown in (Appendix 1),

First, the questionnaire took into account the opinion of the employees about the importance of low back pain in terms of health and socio-economic effects, and whether the impact of persistent low back pain is considered a problem in the employees' opinion that needs to be reduced especially in regard to the psychological and the financial impact.

Secondly, for the motivation of the employees to such a program, we pointed out to the employees what is expected and gained from such a program, especially in the light of social and financial expectations. as this will touch an important area in the future of such employees if they participated in the program, and maybe by participating they would loss the fear of losing their position or jobs in the work market once they are with disability.

Third, the possibility or whether the employees are willing to participate in such program brought to mind that these employees are still under medical treatment or rehabilitations at that moment.

Fourth, tried to obtain a free speech or personal opinion in a professional aspect from the employees regarding whether their organizations are sincerely concerned with helping them to return to work early and by adapting the work place to fit the new possibility of the employees.

The type or rhythm of questions that were asked were in such phrases as "It is important for me to minimize the psychological and financial impacts", "Being absence from work gives me the feeling that I am not part of the organization any more", "If there is such a program that will help me to return to work as early as medically possible by helping me to adapt to my work situation, I would participate in such a program", "I would like to participate in a health program, if that program diminishes my health complain", "being disabled can become a vicious cycle, the longer an employee stays out of the workplace the more difficult it becomes to re-establish the work", " my organization helps me to return to work with my health complain", " my organization will adapt my work situation if necessary", " I will return to work only when I am fully recovered" . Possible answers categories were as such fully agree, agree, fully disagree and disagree.

3.2.2. Selection of respondents

The questionnaire (Appendix 1) was distributed among 50 employees who are working at a private section; their ages ranged between 18- 60 years, and we tried to limit our questionnaire distribution to those who had had medical history of low back pain at some point in their working career. However, it was important for us to also take all the respondents' opinion about how positively they are and their willingness to participate in early return to work program even though they did not have a previous medical history of low back pain.

The distribution of the questionnaires was done either manually or via e-mails. The manually distributed questionnaire were handed over to workers with low back pain coming to the medical committee of the General Organization of the Social Insurance (GOSI), for medical assessment or compensation (usually blue collar worker).

The other group of questionnaires that were distributed via e-mail was sent through the human resource management office of the companies that were pleasantly participating in this study. I also managed to send some emails as well to colleagues and friends whom had medical history of low back pain and of which I knew.

3.3. Employers

Now we come to answering the second part of the study questions:
3. Is there a problem in organizations related to low back pain in Saudi Arabia?
4. Do employers have a positive attitude towards development of early return to work programs?
5. Are the employers willing to implement such a program in their own organizations?

3.3.1. Development of interviews

In order to answer the questions of this study, several interviews were arranged to interview the employers. The use of open questions were chosen in regard to the possibility of the implementation of early return to work program in Saudi Arabia's' private organizations, how positive are the employers towards the development of such a program, and how willingly are the employers to implement such a program in their own organizations.

Part of these open questions inquired about the sickness and absenteeism problem especially the low back pain in particular, and about the Disability Management policy of the organization that supports the employees in their return to work process.

Other parts of the interview were concerned with the opinions of the employers regarding the adaptation of workplace to suite their employees and their new possibilities, and whether it is an importance issue for their organizations.

The open questions of the interviews needed to inquire about what would make employers be motivated to implement such a program in their organizations, further more to inquire about the expectations that the employers would encounter as benefit for them once they agree in implanting such a program, and also about their opinion regarding the advantage of this program as is mentioned above.

In other aspects of the open question, the employers asked about the participation of their employees in such a program and how to convince/ persuade them or motivate them to participate in such a program.

3.3.2. Selection of the respondents

Data were collected after conducting several interviews. The first four interviews were conducted with four employer corporations of big organizations that have employments of at least five hundred employees or more. The reason behind the choice of large organizations is the fact that these organizations have a better human resource capacity in regard to tracking and following all the employees in the organization, and accordingly they will be better prepared candidates to apply the early return to work programs.

These interviews were conducted with Human Resource managers due to the fact that they had a better knowledge about the daily issues and problems of the employees, and they had strong clues or records about absenteeism in general, and low back pain absenteeism particularly. But, before moving to the last or fifth interview, a very short and brief words about each of the four organizations should be given.

The first interview was conducted with Human Resource manager of the Riadaa Group (Riadaa is one of the leading companies in the fields of Services Industry, taking a serious role in developing the Services Market in the Saudi Arabia and the region. Also, it is one of the biggest companies in Saudi Arabia in the field of mail delivery, and out-sources).

The second conducted interview was with the Human Resource manager of ORACLE corporation (is specializes in developing and marketing enterprise software products, particularly database management systems. Through organic growth and a number of high-profile acquisitions, Oracle enlarged its share of the software market. By 2007 Oracle ranked third on the list of largest software companies in the world, after Microsoft and IBM).

Interview number three was with Human Resource manager of SKAB Group (one of the largest private sector business groups in the Kingdom of Saudi Arabia with a variety of interconnected business enterprises, spanning such disciplines as Environment Protection & Recycling, Mineral Water Bottling Plant, Contracting, Real Estate, Hospitality Industry, Shopping Malls, Travel & Tourism, Food Products and Construction and Maintenance).

The fourth interview was conducted with Human Resource manager of RAJHI STEEL company (specialized in producing different types of steel products covering about 35% of the Saudi market needs in both commercial and Rebar steel, also covering the international markets through exporting to Gulf Cooperation Council, as well as to some neighboring countries).

I was privileged to have the fifth interview with a human resource consultant who works at one of the human resource consultancy companies. The decision of interviewing a human resource Consultant came to me after interviewing the four Human Resource managers who gave the same opinion; their opinion will be mentioned in the following next chapter. By interviewing a human resource Consultant, I hoped to gain a different point of view. This point of view gets its importance from the consultancy professionalism and experience with different organizations.

The interview done was with one of human resource consultants and who is the owner of a Special Direction Company (Human Resource Consultancy & Recruitment Company, established by group of human resource professionals, both local and international, from various back grounds who complement each other to form a very special team).

3.4. Social Insurance organization

Study questions:
   6. Is the cost of the low back pain a problem for the social insurance organization?
   7. Do social insurance policy makers think that early return to work programs could be cost saving?
   8. Are social insurance policy makers willing to support the implementation of such a program?
   9. Do social insurance policy makers think that the employees and employers will support such a program?

3.4.1. Development of interviews

The modalities to answer the study questions were based on conducting interviews using open questions that focus on and are concerned with the possibility of implementation of early return to work program for the employee with low back pain in Saudi Arabia.

The open question had concerns with the social insurance policy maker opinions regarding the early return to work program; cost saving for social insurance was a definite matter to attend to, and whether the social insurance organization are wiling to participate at all in such a program.

The open questions of the interviews were intended to find out about the cost problem of the social insurance especially costs due to low back pain sickness absence and compensation.

From a different perspective the open questions inquired as well about the conditions and the desire to support and motivate the early return to work program by the social insurance.

Also the questions of the interview had without doubt to have a light shed on the perspective of the social insurance policy maker about the willingness of the employees to participate in such a program and about the willingness of the employers to adapt the work place to the new needs of their employees and to participate in such a program.

3.4.2. Selection of the respondents

Answering the third or last part of the study questions (6th, 7th, 8th, 9th question) needed interviews to be done with two decision makers in the social insurance organization in order to collect the required data.

First decision maker to be interviewed was the vice governor for insurance affair of the General Organization for Social Insurance. While the second decision maker to be interviewed was with the general manager of medical department and the head of the medical committees of the General Organization for Social Insurance.

In the following text, we will give a very short brief word about the General Organization for Social Insurance in Saudi Arabia as an explanatory paragraph of the system.

The General Organization for Social Insurance (GOSI) was established to apply social insurance rules and implement its regulation, particularly, concerning achieving the lawfully social coverage, collecting contributions from employers and paying benefits to entitled insured persons or their family members. GOSI is a semi-state body that has its independent financial and administrative entity supervised by a board of directors consisting of eleven members; the Minister of Labor (Chairman), GOSI Governor (Vice Chairman), three members representing Ministry of Labor, Ministry of Finance and Ministry of Health, three insured members highly qualified in their business, and three members of employers. Activities of GOSI are practiced within its Head Office and twenty four field offices distributed allover the Kingdom's provinces and districts. The Social Insurance Law is a form of social solidarity and cooperation that the society provides for its citizens and provides social protection to the private sector workers as well as a category of workers in the public sector in order to provide a good life for the workers and their families after termination of employment due to retirement, disability or death. It also provides medical care for occupational injuries and diseases as well as the required compensations in case of occupational disability or death (GOSI, 2009).

3.5. Data analysis

The data analysis in this study had two parts; the quantitative study, displayed the percentages from the distributed questionnaire on to the employees. The second part, the qualitative study was obtained from the in-depth interviews with the employers and the social insurance organization policy makers.

4. Results

This chapter will display the data and the results from the study. First, the descriptive data will be presented for the employees, subsequently for employers and at the end the Social Insurance Organization.

4.1. Employees

Study questions:
1. Do employees with low back pain have a positive attitude towards early return to work programs?
2. Are employees with low back pain willing to participate in such a program?

4.1.1. Characteristics of the respondents

50 questionnaires were distributed over to different workplaces, only 43 workers out of the 50 were considered as respondents, out of which 33 workers of the 43 respondents had given history of low back pain, and although the other ten respondents did not have pervious medical history of low back pain but we took all the respondent opinion in consideration because this study is about the feasibility of implementation of the program.

Table 1: Characteristic of the study group of employees (N=43)

Characteristic	Number	Percentage
Gender		
Male	35	81.4%
Female	8	18.6%
Age		
< 31	6	13.9%
31 – 40	11	25.6%
41 – 50	18	41.9%
51- 60	8	18.6%
Occupational status		
Blue collar worker	27	62.8%
White collar worker	16	37.2

The results and data which are presented in (Table 1) show the characteristic of the 43 respondents. It also shows gender differences, the percentage at different ages, as well as the occupational status of the employees.

The study group of 43 respondents with history of low back pain consisted of 35 male (81.4%) and eight female (18.6), age of the respondent were between (31 – 60 years), while the majority had the age between (41 -50) years, and the majority of the respondents were the blue collar worker showing the percentage of (62.8 %).

4.1.2. Employees' attitude towards LBP and ERTW programs

In order to answer the first study question, the results and data from the employees' questionnaire (presented in table 2) displayed how the employees judge low back pain as a problem and it also showed that they are positive and self-confident about the advantages of the program.

Table 2 showed that the majority of the respondents experienced low back pain as a health problem (83.8%) and as a socio-economic problem (76.8 %). Also a majority of respondents (93%) saw the importance of minimizing the psychological and financial impacts of low back pain.

Also Table 2 displayed that the majority of the respondents agreed about the financial motivation of the early return to work program by returning the income to its pre injury level (95.4%). While most of the respondents de-motivated for a return to work program when they had early retirement (55.8%).

On the other hand, majority of the respondents experience social advantage of early return to work program and how that such program can give the employees the feeling of being still part of the organization (79.1%). feeling of contributing the skills (65.2%). The study showed that the majority of the respondents (90.7 %) agreed to the difficulty to re-establish the work for an employee who stayed out of the workplace for longer periods of time.

Table 2: Employees attitude towards LBP and RTW.

Questions	Fully agree	Agree	Disagree	Fully disagree
For me persistent low back pain is a major health problem	15 (34.9%)	21 (48.9%)	6 (13.9%)	1 (2.3%)
For me persistent low back pain is a major socio-economic problem	14 (32.6%)	19 (44.2%)	8 (18.6%)	2 (4.7%)
It is important for me to minimize the psychological and financial impacts	14 (32.5%)	26 (60.5%)	3 (7%)	0 (0%)
Most injured workers can return to some type of work even while they are still recovering.	6 (13.9%)	15 (34.9%)	18 (41.9%)	4 (9.3%)
When I have an early retirement or illness retirement I will not be motivated for a return to work program.	8 (18.6%)	11 (25.6%)	23 (53.5%)	1 (2.3%)
The sooner an employees returns to work, the sooner her or his income will return to its pre-injury level	19 (44.2%)	22 (51.2%)	2 (4.6%)	0 (0%)
Being disabled can become a vicious cycle, The longer an employee stays out of the workplace the more difficult it becomes to re-establish the work.	26 (60.5%)	13 (30.2%)	4 (9.3%)	0 (0%)
Being absence from work gives me the feeling that I am not part of the organization any more.	16 (37.2%)	18 (41.9%)	7 (16.3%)	2 (4.6%)
The feeling of contributing the skills and abilities to the whole will be lost as long as employee stays off work	18 (41.9%)	10 (23.3%)	12 (27.9%)	3 (7%)

4.1.3. Willingness of the employees to participate in ERTW program

In order to answer the second study question, the results and data of the employees' questionnaire which are presented in (Table 3) displays the willingness of employees regarding the participation in early return to work program.

The results and data presented in (Table 3) display that all of the respondents (100 %) showed their willingness to participate in a program that diminishes their health complain, even though such a program will return them to work early by helping them to adapt to the work situation and to adapt the work place according to their possibility. Most of the respondents showed their ability to work with their health complain (74.4%), if the program supported them to return to workplace situation (86.1%).

However, the majority of the respondents (79.1%) showed that they are unwilling to return to work if they are not fully recovered, and most of them disagreed (58.2%) that the workers had to return to work as soon as possible.

Table 3 showed that the majority of the respondents' experienced an unhelpfulness of the organization (67.5 %) in returning to work early, and (60.5 %) saw the unwillingness of the organization to adapt the workplace for the employee possibility if necessary. while (65.1%) agreed that the return to work is possible when the workplace is adapted or modified to their possibility.

On other hand, most of the respondents saw the difficulty of returning to (83.7%) work after a long period of sickness or absence which increases the threshold to return to work (67.4%).

Table 3: Employees' willingness to participate in RTW

Questions	Fully agree	Agree	Disagree	Fully disagree
Being absent from work for a long a period increase the threshold to return to work.	6 (13.9%)	23 (53.5%)	8 (18.6%)	3 (7%)
I will return to work only when I am fully recovered.	16 (37.2%)	18 (41.9%)	9 (20.9%)	0 (0%)
Worker with low back pain have to return to work as soon as medically possible.	2 (4.6%)	16 (37.2%)	22 (51.2%)	3 (7%)
If there is a program that will help me to return to work as early as medically possible by helping me to adapt to my work situation, I would participate in such a program.	34 (79.1%)	9 (20.9%)	0 (0%)	0 (0%)
After a long period of sickness absence, I find it difficult to return to work.	19 (44.2%)	17 (39.5%)	5 (11.6%)	2 (4.7%)
I would prefer a program that supports me to return to workplace situation.	16 (37.2%)	21 (48.9%)	6 (13.9%)	0 (0%)
Return to work is possible when the workplace is adapted to my possibility.	5 (11.6%)	23 (53.5%)	15 (34.9%)	0 (0%)
I have health complain but I am able to work.	13 (30.2%)	19 (44.2%)	8 (18.6%)	3 (7%)
My organization helps me to return to work with my health complain.	2 (4.6%)	12 (27.9%)	26 (60.5%)	3 (7%)
My organization will adapt my work situation if necessary.	2 (4.6%)	15 (34.9%)	20 (46.5%)	6 (14%)
I would like to participate in a health program if it helps me to return to work earlier.	21 (48.8%)	18 (41.9%)	4 (9.3%)	0 (0%)
I would like to participate in a health program if that program diminishes my health complain.	27 (62.8%)	16 (37.2%)	0 (0%)	0 (0%)

4.2. Employers

Study questions:
3. Is there a problem in organizations related to low back pain in Saudi Arabia?
4. Do employers have a positive attitude towards development of early return to work programs?
5. Are the employers willing to implement such a program in their own organizations?

4.2.1. Problem of Sickness absenteeism due to low back pain and RTW policy

Interviews were held with four employers, all interviewees agreed that low back pain is considered a problem of sickness and absenteeism in their organizations. All the four interviews with the employers indicated that lower back pain does indeed lower the productivity and negatively affects the profitability.

Most of them did not have an account of the effect of this problem on the economic measures (factors) of the organization; the only employer that had measured the influence of this phenomenon is (Riadaa). The management estimated that low back pain problems decreased the productivity by 15% in the year 2007. Furthermore, it caused a 4% decrease in profitability as a result of work delay.

As much as the employers did like the idea during the interview however, none of them did have any written policy in their organization in supporting the employees in their returning to work, but sometimes they did try to help the employees to return to work by trying to change his or her work, or by decreasing the work load, and that somehow depended first of all on the decision of the general manager or the owner/s. For instance, the human resource manager of SKAB group said *"in my department we try to help our employees by collecting information about his/her medical situation and what are their new situations requirement in work place, and then send it to the one who have the decision in such situations"*.

And second of all on different factors can affect the general manager or the owner/s decision, like the employees working position, working experience, the knowledge, the employees relationship with the customers or the agents and depending on his or her regular working evaluations (every three month or every six month or annually depending on each organization). That means that the worker who is not of much benefit to the organization would sacrifice losing his/her position to a new recruitment. Another important factor manifests in the social factors that can lead the organization to keep employees just for social reasons.

4.2.2. Positive attitude towards development of early return to work program

All human resource mangers agreed that helping the sick employees to return to work early as soon as possible can be a high priority for their organizations, as this defiantly decreases the need to pay overtimes to get the work that was normally performed by workers who are absent, and will reduce the costs of recruiting as well as training new employees to replace sick workers, and that may increase staff loyalty.

Retaining experience is also a major issue for these companies. The activity of a company is affected to a great extent by using the retained experience as a policy. For example ORACLE Corporation as a software developer that depends mainly on intellectual capital considers retaining knowledge and experience as a major priority. The human resource manager of the company mentioned that *"even in case of absenteeism, the company can provide the employee with a PC, and internet connection and he/she can work from home"*.

The Human Resource Consultant gave the same positive opinion regarding early return to work program, and that much of the benefit can be gained for the organizations through implementing such a program, which may lead to a decrease in their sickness absenteeism problem, and reduce the cost incurred by the organizations by employees' absence. On the other hand, the Human Resource Consultant elucidated that the most important benefit from this program would be the retaining of experiences which as he believed is the most important for the organizations.

4.2.3. Willingness to implement ERTW program

During the interviews that were conducted, a semi-presentation or explanation of what early return to work program would be like and what benefits for both employers and employees would gain from implementing such a program was given. After the presentation, the question of whether they are willing and /or interested to participate in such a program. All of the four employers gave the same answer, that they would participate in such a program only if it were made obligatory by The Ministry of Labor, because the current Labor Law book of policies doesn't contain any kind of obligation that would lead them to apply such a program. Thus, the decision is kept in the hands of the employers (i.e. it's up to the employer to decide if they want to keep an employee and to early return them back to work by adapting the workplace or whether wanting to fire the employee). For instance the human resource manager of Riadaa Company said *"the participation of my organization in such program is easier said than done, if there is nothing in the labor law that means the decision is made only by the owner"*.

Asking about the employee's capacity and desire to participate in the program, the employers stated that the employees will participate, if he/she is well educated about the program, and more aware of its benefits. On the other hand, negative rewards (i.e. punishments) can be taken against him/her in case of refusing to participate. These punishments can take many forms for example, salary discounts, demotion, and negative evaluation reports. From their experiences, human resource managers in Riadaa and Rajhi Steel Company stated, however, that the best strategy for dealing with this issue is the pay discount. The four interviewees indicated that the companies do not have a positive reward policy; they rather use negative rewards as the major policy.

On the other hand, the Human Resource Consultant gave a different opinion. This is due to his experience in consulting different organizations and dealing with different owners. In addition, he is outside the boarders of the company, so he has a better view than the people who are inside the company. When he was asked the same question regarding the willingness of the employers to participate in an early return to work program, he thought that such a program can be applied by the employers if they were rewarded by applying this program. In other words, the key is to motivate the employers to apply such a program, and not by mere forcing them to apply such program by adding articles in the Labor Law because there are some articles in the Labor Law that are not followed by some employer, for instance he gave the following article which are written in the Saudi Arabian Labor Law:

"If a worker sustains a work injury that results in a loss in his usual capabilities that does not prevent him from performing another job, the employer, in whose service the work injury was sustained, shall employ said worker in a suitable job for the wage specified for such job. This shall not prejudice the workers compensation for the injury" (Labor Law in Saudi Arabia).

"Each employer employing twenty- five workers or more where the nature of his work allows recruitment of the professionally disabled shall employ a number of disabled that represents at least 4% of the total number of his workers whether through nomination by the employment units or otherwise, and he shall send to the competent labor office a list of the jobs and posts occupied by the professionally rehabilitated disabled persons and their wages" (Labor Law in Saudi Arabia).

The Human Resource Consultant thought that the previous articles are not applied in reality due to the absence of sanctions on the organization that did not apply it. To implement such a program we need in addition to the sanction, a reward system that provides incentives to the employers who applied the early return to work program which can take different forms, and he gave the following ideas: decreasing the social insurance payment paid by the employers' side (the total social insurance payment equals to 18% of the employers wages, 9% paid by the employers and the other 9% paid by the employees), decreasing the occupational hazard insurance which is also paid by employers (equals to 2% of employees wages), and/ or to increase the Ministry Labor approval of the recruitment from abroad for the purpose of work.

4.3. Social Insurance Organization

Study questions:

6. Is the cost of the low back pain a problem for the social insurance organization?
7. Do social insurance policy makers think that early return to work programs could be cost saving?
8. Are social insurance policy makers willing to support the implementation of such a program?
9. Do social insurance policy makers think that the employees and employers will support such a program?

4.3.1. Cost problem of low back pain

The interview with the Social Insurance policy makers showed that low back pain is considered as a cost problem for the social insurance organization because, complaints will increase the cost of ill health retirements or early retirement and the compensation claims. The general manager of medical department - head of the medical committees of the General Organization for Social Insurance does not, hold the knowledge about the real cost due to his technical specialization as a medical doctor.

The vice governor for insurance affair of the General Organization for Social Insurance had a broader vision due to his position in the top management level in the organization. He saw that the cost will be reduced if applying such a policy, and he estimated that about 27% of the work related injuries are related to low back problem, and this costs the organization about 1.7% of the total costs.

4.3.2. Positive attitude towards development of early return to work program

Both of the interviewees were positive about the early return to work program and agreed about the benefit that can be gained from the program for the social insurance organization in addition to both the employees and the employers.

The general manager of medical department - head of the medical committees of the General Organization for Social Insurance had in fact an experience with this program, and he shared with us his own personal practice with his patients of a low back pain, and how the early return to work program made the workers recover faster, and he strongly agreed that such a program can indeed decrease the sickness absence and the need for post-treatment work restrictions. He also agreed that the program decreases the percentage of disability and speeds up the recovery, not to mention restoring labor force participation and reducing the negative financial impacts of disability, and decrease the expenditure of sickness and disability benefit which as mentioned earlier are considered as cost problem for the social insurance organization. As he said *"I know well from my experience and my work positions what the medical and the financial advantages are. Especially for the employees who's are the most important group to us and I am always asking for the cooperation of the hospitals in order to return our employees back to work as soon as possible and stopping the unnecessary sick leaves that are given by treating physicians".*

On other hand, the vice governor for insurance affairs of the General Organization for Social Insurance had no experience with early return to work program. Nevertheless, he agreed that such a program can reduce financial impacts of the disability for both the employers and the employees who are willing to participate in such a program.

4.3.3. Willingness to support the implementation of ERTW program

Both of the interviewees confirmed the willingness of the social insurance organization to support the implementation of the program in Saudi Arabia. However, both of them gave different opinion about the difficulty in the implementation of this program.

The general manager of medical department - head of the medical committees illuminated the willingness of the social insurance organization to support the implementation of the program, but he saw that it would be difficult to implement such a program in Saudi Arabia through social insurance organization, because he thought that implementing such a program needs strong cooperation between the organization, the hospital, and the social insurance organizations, which does not exist these days. Furthermore, he saw the necessity of having an occupational physician for each organization or at least for a group of organizations. The occupational physician, in his opinion, plays an important role in qualifying the worker for his/her new duties and in helping the organization arrange the job requirements for the employee after returning back. He also stressed on the importance of educating "treating physicians" about the early return to work program (i.e., the medical benefit, and when to intervene by applying such program as a treatment).

The vice governor for insurance affairs of the General Organization for Social Insurance was in favor of this program, and he also illuminated the willingness of the social insurance organization to support the implementation of the program. But, on the other hand, he stated a number of hurdles that blocked the proper implementation of the program in Saudi Arabia.

First, there is a deficiency in trained personnel in this field. That's why; the organization follows the policy of expanding the education base by providing scholarships abroad in educational organizations renowned for their work-related scientific programs.

Second, it would be difficult to make the organizations participate in such a program, because the General Organization for Social Insurance is an insurance organization and does not have the authority to implement the early return to work program. He believed that implementation of such a program needs to be part of the labor law and watch how it is applied by employers. This authority, meanwhile, belongs to the Ministry of Labor and not the General Organization for Social Insurance.

Third, the lack of cooperation between the social insurance organization and the employer in planning for and applying early return to work program is another problem.

4.3.4. Possibility to participate in ERTW program for employees and employers

Both interviewees explained the simplicity of participation of the employees in the program because the program is based on the best interest of the employees especially from the health and financial perspective; while it showed difficulty in the participation of the employers because usually the employers seek their own financial aspect. When asked the general manager of medical department, if the employees would show willingness to participate in such program, he thought that they will participate in the program if the treating physician and the occupational physician clarified to them the benefit that they will gain from their participation. And when asked if the employers showed any willingness to participate, he explained the difficulty in the employers participation due to the difficulty in convincing them about the importance of such a program in reducing the cost of sickness absenteeism due to low back pain, this situation points out the importance of the creation of rules to regulate such program in each organization.

When asked the vice governor if the employee's were willing to participate in such a program, he believed that their willingness is related to the degree of their knowledge about the benefits of such a program, and another important factor is the personality of the employee. Some employees prefer not to return back to work until they are sure that they have completely recovered, while others do not have a big problem in this regard. The vice governor believed that employers' adaptation of work place to suit the employee's new possibility depends mainly on the estimated economic benefit for reintegrating the employee. But, on the other hand, he saw that these organizations should have a social responsibility commitment that would enable them to reconsider their priorities (i.e. they can replace the economic benefit for social morale among employees in the organization).

"Owners of the private organizations should be educated about their social commitment in order to participate in such a program" vice governor.

5. Conclusion, discussion and recommendations

The previous chapters provided us with the results that were obtained from the data collected during this study. In this chapter, we will first give you an idea about the limitations (5.1.) of this study where by knowing it, we can go to the conclusions (5.2.) of the result in order to answer the study questions that were stated in chapter two, then the discussion (5.3.) and the recommendations (5.4.) will be displayed subsequently.

5.1. Limitations

The lack of knowledge of what and how to implement the ERTW program on both sides of the employees and the employers from different sectors of the work market made it frustrating at first, let alone the time needed to put out presentations explanations and discussions.

In this study we had questionnaires distributed to employees, interviews with Human resource managers and the social insurance organization policy makers. Perhaps, if we distributed a larger number of questionnaire it might have given a wider scope in order to understand the needs and opinions of more people; and by doing a study on a specific age group with low back pain or a study on a sub group of employees with the same low back pain in a specific period of time; even arranging more interviews with employers and additional interview with the owners of organizations/ companies. We have to admit that we should have included small organizations as well, as their needs and opinions for implementing the program may differ from big organizations as those that were included in our study.

The study in this book was a general approach and it would have been more feasible if it was combined with a statistical analysis about low back pain in Saudi Arabia to give a stronger reinforcement to our study.

The limited number of published studies on low back pain and disability in Saudi Arabia made it difficult to know the true size of the problem in Saudi Arabia. That is why whenever we needed data we had to obtain it from each organization separately.

5.2. Conclusion

Knowing the previous limitations, we can conclude about the feasibility of implementing the early return to work program for employees with low back pain in Saudi Arabia is possible but needs a lot of effort and change from the three groups of the study, the employees, employers and social insurance organization.

We can conclude that the low back pain sicknesses and absenteeism is cost consuming for the employer and the social insurance organization, as the cost is estimated to be 4% decrease in the profitability of the employer and is going to cost the social insurance organization 1.7% of the total cost.

The employees had a positive attitude in relation to the program and showed willingness to participate in such a program if implemented. However, there was an obstacle, where it was clear that most of employees will not participate until they have full medical recovery and not when they are under medical treatment. This in conclusion was the same prospective that the social insurance organization policy makers had.

The employers had a positive attitude in relation to the program. But, since the employers are seeking the fastest financial benefit, they are not in favor of social commitment or expenditure for implementing specific program by specifying a new budget and hiring special staff working on this program. Hence, they have no interest in developing a written policy in their organization for such programs. This conclusion goes hand in hand with the perspectives of the social insurance organization policy makers about the participation of employers in such a program. Let's not forget that the employees do know that their employers are not interested in helping them to return to work early or to change the work place to the employees' new possibility.

The social insurance organization knew in fact that it cannot persuade the employers to implement such a program due to the absence of an authority.

On other hand, we can conclude from the previous results from the interviews with the employers and the social insurance organizations policy makers, that the implementation of early return to work program in private organizations in Saudi Arabia should be obligatory from related governmental organizations. For example, the Ministry of Labor, by editing some regulation regarding the ERTW program to labor law.

Also we can conclude that the imposition of the program by forcing it is not the only solution, that due to some written articles in the labor law that are not followed by some organizations. The reason behind this disobedience may be due to the absence of financial rewards for the employers and motivation. That's why the implementation of the ERTW program in Saudi Arabia needs to have motivation in addition to the editing of the regulation in the Labor Law.

Social insurance organization policy makers, think that early return to work programs can decrease the rate of disability and this is going to be cost saving especially for the social insurance organization and the employer. However, that may be true; they are still aware and sure of the support they will get from the employees but not from the employers regarding the implementation of this program.

Finally, based on the positive thinking of the employees, the employers and the social insurance organization policy makers and the knowledge of the cost consumption for sickness and absenteeism of employees with low back pain, it would be good to start the implementation of the program in Saudi Arabia, taking into account, some recommendations that will be mentioned later on.

5.3. Discussion

Based on collected data and results, there is a possibility of implementing the ERTW program in Saudi Arabian organizations after doing some modifications and changes in the disability management policy of the organizations and in the labor law. But, there are some controversies from the opinions of both the employees and the employers.

The results of questionnaire we obtained from the workers/ employees showed that the employees are convinced about the importance of the program from the financial and the psychological point of view. But, not from the medical or health aspect, as a large sector of employees prefers not to return to work until they are fully recovered. This point is in direct relationship with the employees who's refused returning to work as soon as medically possible, and this is why health issue has to be re-looked at if we are going to implement the program. It is worthwhile to know that majority of people in Saudi Arabia are totally convinced that a person with low back pain should have bed rest. Having said that, we find it surprising that other employees are keen to implement ERTW program because they would reach their previous monthly salary back to the way it was before having the disability as well as the feel of being part of the organization and to share the responsibility once again with his/ her co-workers.

Moving to the next step of the willingness of the employees to participate in this program; it appears possible (according to their opinions). But, majority will probably not participate; this is due to several reasons: they see that a worker with low back pain needs his rest until full recovery (as mentioned earlier). Another reason is, the sense that most organizations (especially the ones that the respondents work at) are not going to do much change to adapt to its employees new situation or needs to motivate them to early return to work, as one of the employers indicated by saying *"why should I return to work for an organization that does not care"*.

On the other hand, the employees whom were granted their early retirement as a consequence of a disability are not in favor to implement such a program for several reasons, most importantly is the fact that they will no longer be motivated to return to work early, if at all, as they are already getting used to their new life style and their new retirement salary and therefore are not willing to take any step to change it. In other words, not in favor of implementing ERTW program.

Another reason may be that they see it as a viscous cycle from their perspective; that is to say, the longer you stay out of the workplace, the harder or more difficult it becomes to re-establish the work. Some respondents agreed that it had a direct relationship that being absence from work for long periods is going to increase the threshold of RTW.

It was found that the employers had a positive attitude regarding the ERTW program and its many advantages, and benefits, and this is because they are aware of the increasing number of sicknesses and absenteeism due to low back pain in their organizations. However, none of the employers were keen enough to participate in it for a number of reasons. The reasons may be due to the fact that the interviews were not arranged with the owners, instead the interviews were with the human resource managers that were very diplomatic in their answers to give a good impression on how the company is willing to accept to new programs, and at the same time they could not give clear answers because there is no written policy and the fact that any final decision is kept in the hands of the owner.

Finding similar or matching response from most human resource managers, lead to seek a different response which found in the interview had with the human resource consultant. Another reason is the unawareness of company owners of how programs like ERTW program can decrease the cost expenditure on absenteeism due to low back pain.

5.4. Recommendations

There is a mixture of feelings about ERTW program in Saudi Arabia. This mixture of feelings is for both the employees as well as the employers. Therefore, we have to strengthen the positive feeling for all groups of this study and decrease the obstacles behind implementing such a program.

Another thing to remember is that, the early return work program is not a computer system and that it will and should differ from one ill worker to another depending on his or her possibility.

A good start is to educate both the employees and the employers about the ERTW program. This is a big important step in order to teach them about the possibilities when implementing such a program; education can take different modalities. An example is to arrange small talks or setting up semi-seminars on monthly base; Setting up information websites can speed up the process for learning about the program especially when it focuses on the benefits for both parties; Courses or diplomas for educating occupational physicians and treating physicians can be another modality of education, and educating privet companies and organizations about the support and contribution to the community is mandatory and can be displayed by reintegrating employees or even giving support.

Another recommendation is to have a rewarding system for those who are keen to implement the ERTW program; different forms of reward can take place as decreasing the social insurance payment paid by the employers' side, or by decreasing the occupational hazard insurance which is also paid by employers.

I also recommend finding or creating new working opportunities for the employees with the new possibility in numerous sectors of the work market to meet the needs of the employees; having bonus payments given to the participating employees is also a reward system as this will defiantly rest their minds from the fear of losing the jobs they once occupied.

Initiating any new project or program will have it fears at first, that's why we can recommend implementing the ERTW program in two model organizations to be studied and to get monthly feedback.

Giving support or grants to employers in order to decrease the costs that they would bear when implementing the program, as the employee returning early to work is still under recovery and is still unable to give full performance. Grants can help as well in adapting a new work possibility. The disabled employee may also be given a bonus in addition to his/her monthly salary as they tend to being paid less (as in the UK).

Cooperation between the social insurance organization, the employers and the hospital is strongly recommended to ensure a better chance for implementing the ERTW program. Indeed the cooperation need to be increased especially between the social insurance organization with the employers, and the hospitals with employers. Hence, there is good cooperation between the social insurance organization with the hospitals as a result from the interview of the medical director of the social insurance organization.

Laying out a written policy and regulations of ERTW program can help employees of large and low pay salaries working in either large or small organization to know their benefits and their rights.

Assigning an occupational physician for each large corporation and/or one for a group of small organization can help especially when they have been educated well about the ERTW program because, the task of an occupation physician assigned in most organizations today is to mainly diagnose the compensation and then asses the degree of disability.

Appendix A:

Employees' questionnaire

1. **Age**: _____ years

2. **Gender**:   1) Male   2) Female

3. **Type of job**:   1) office work   2) manual work

4. **Work experience**: _____ years

5. **Do you have medical history of low back pain?**
    1) Yes   2) No

6. **Have you ever had sick leaves due to low back pain?**
    1) Yes   2) No
   a. In case of "yes" go to question 7&8.

7. **What was the maximum period of sick leaves you had due to low back pain?** _____ days

8. **Number of sick leaves per years due low back pain**: _____

Questions	Fully agree	Agree	Disagree	Fully disagree
For me persistent low back pain is a major health problem				
For me persistent low back pain is a major socio-economic problem				
It is important for me to minimize the psychological and financial impacts				
Most injured workers can return to some type of work even while they are still recovering.				
When I have an early retirement or illness retirement I will be not motivated for a return to work programs.				
The sooner an employees returns to work, the sooner her or his income will return to its pre-injury level				
Being disabled can become a vicious cycle, The longer an employee stays out of the workplace the more difficult it becomes to re-establish the work.				
Being absence from work for a long a period increase the threshold for return to work				
Being absence from work gives me the feeling that I am not part of the organization any more.				
The feeling of contributing the skills and abilities to the whole will be lost as long as employee stays off work				
I will return to work only when I am fully recovered.				
Worker with low back pain have to return to work as soon as medically possible				

If there is a program that will help me to return to work early as medically possible by helping me to adapt to my work situation, I would participate at such program				
After a long period of sickness absence, I find it difficult to return to work.				
I would prefer a program that supporting me to return to workplace situation				
Return to work is possible when the workplace is adapted to my possibility				
I have health complain but I am able to work				
My organization helps me to return to work with my health complain				
My organization will adapt my work situation if necessary				
I would like to participate at health program if that help me return to work earlier				
I would like to participate at health program if that program diminish my health complain				

Appendix B:

Checklist interview with employers

- Is low back pain considered a problem of sickness and absenteeism in your organization? Explain how.
- Is there a policy in the organization that supports employees in their return to work process? And how it is organized?
- Do you think that helping the patient to return to work as soon as medically possible can be a high priority for your organization? Why?
- Do you think that being at work in an adaptive situation is healthy for the organization?
- What do you think about such a program, will it decrease the need to pay overtime to get work normally performed by workers who are absent?
- Do you think that the costs of recruiting and training new employees to replace injured/ill workers are going to be reduced by implementing such a program?
- What do you think about your employees, are they willing to participate in such a program?
- Do you have any experience with such a program & what is your opinion?
- Will you participate in such a program if such a program will help the employees with low back pain to return to workplace as soon as possible?
- Would you ask or motivate your employees to participate in such a program?
- Would you adapt the workplace for those employees?
- Do you think that applying such a program to the organization will increase staff loyalty?
- Do you have a DM program or any similar program in your organization?

Appendix C:

Checklist interview with social insurance policy makers

- Is low back pain considered as a cost problem for the social insurance organization? Can you give some information about the cost?
- Do you think that the cost of ill health retirement or early retirement and compensation claims for low back pain is going to be reduced by implementing an early return to work program?
- Do you think the sickness absence and the need for post-treatment work restrictions will be decreased by an early return to work program?
- Do you think it possible to implement such a program in Saudi Arabia?
- Would the social insurance organization support or motivate the implementation of such a program?
- Do you have any experience with such a program & what is your opinion?
- Do you think that the employees are willing to participate in such a program?
- Do you think that the employees are willing to return to work as soon as medically possible?
- Under what conditions (reasons) do you think employers are willing to adapt the work palace to diminish the risk to low back pain?
- Do you think that employers are willing to implement such a program?

References:

1. Al-Arfaj Abdurrahman S., Salman S. Al-Saleh, Suliman R. Alballa, Abdullah N. Al-Dalaan, Sultan A. Bahabri, Mohammed A. Al-Sekeit, Mohammed A. Mousa, *How common is back pain in Al-Qaseem region* . Saudi Med J 2003; Vol. 24 (2): 170-173.
2. Anema JR, Steenstra IA, Urlings IJ, Bongers PM, de Vroome EM, van Mechelen W. Participatory *ergonomics as a return-to-work intervention: a future challenge?* Am J Ind Med. 2003;44:273–281.
3. Anema JR, Steenstra IA, Bongers PM, de Vet HCW, Knol DL, van Mechelen W. *Multidisciplinary Rehabilitation for Subacute Low Back Pain: Graded Activity or Workplace Intervention or Both? A Randomized Controlled Trial.* Spine. 2007;32:291–298.
4. Bratton, J., & Gold, J. (2007). *Human Resource Management. Theory and practice.* Palgrave Macmillan.
5. Devereaux, M., *Low Back Pain,* Medical Clinics of North Americ; Volume 93, Issue 2 (March 2009).
6. De Jong AM, Vink P. *Participatory ergonomics applied in installation work.* Appl Ergon. 2002;33:439–448.
7. Frank J, Sinclair S, Hogg-Johnson S, Shannon H, Bombardier C, Beaton D, Cole D., *preventing disability from work-related low-back pain, new evidence gives new hope if we can just get all the players onside*, CMAJ 1998; 158(12): 1625-1631.
8. GOSI, General Organization for Social Insurance, www.gosi.gov.sa, 10-7-2009.
9. Hansen A, Edlund C, Bränholm IB., Significant resources needed for return to work after sick leave. Work. 2005;25(3):231-40.
10. Hildebrandt, Jan; Pfingsten, Michael; Saur, Petra; Jansen, Jürgen,(1997). *Prediction of Success from a Multidisciplinary Treatment Program for Chronic Low Back Pain.* Spine 22, 990-1001.
11. Hoogendoorn, W. E., et al., *High physical work load and low job satisfaction increase the risk of sickness absence due to low back pain: results of a prospective cohort study.* Occup Environ Med, 2002. 59(5)
12. Hunter1, Nicola. *Chris Sharp2, Julie Denning3 and Lutgen Terblanche1, Evaluation of a functional restoration programmed in chronic low back pain,* Occupational Medicine, 11 August 2006;56:497–500.

13. Kärrholm J, Ekholm K, Ekholm J, Bergroth A, Ekholm KS., *Systematic cooperation between employer, occupational health service and social insurance office: a 6-year follow-up of vocational rehabilitation for people on sick-leave, including economic benefits.* J Rehabil Med. 2008 Aug; 40(8):628-36.
14. Koopman FS, Edelaar M, Slikker R, Reynders K, van der Woude LH, Hoozemans MJ., *effectiveness of a Multidisciplinary Occupational Training Program for Chronic Low Back Pain: A Prospective Cohort Study*, Am J Phys Med Rehabil., Volume 83(2), February 2004, pp 94-103
15. Labor Law in Saudi Arabia, Ministry of labor: www.mol.gov.sa, 15-5-2009
16. Loisel P, Abenhaim L, Durand P, Esdaile JM, Suissa S, Gosselin L, Simard R, Turcotte J, Lemaire J. *A population-based, randomized clinical trial on back pain management.* Spine. 1997;22:2911–2918.
17. Mayer T, Smith S, Keeley J, Tabor J, Bovasso E, Gatchel RJ., *Quantification of lumbar function: II. Sagittal plane trunk strength in chronic low back pain patients.* Spine 1985;10:765–72.
18. Mayer T, Gatchel RJ, Mayer H, Kishino ND, Keeley J, Mooney V. A., prospective two-year study of functional restoration in industrial low back injury: An objective assessment procedure. JAMA 1987;258.
19. Merskey, H.. *Pain terms: a list with definitions and notes on usage.* Pain 1979, 6:249-252.
20. Millington, M.J., & Strauser, D.R. (1998). *Planning strategies in disability management.* Work, Volume 10, Number 3, May 1998, pp. 261-270(10).
21. Molde Hagen E, Grasdal A, Eriksen HR, *Does early intervention with a light mobilization program reduce long-term sick leave for low back pain: a 3-year follow-up study*, pine (Phila Pa 1976). 2004 Oct 15;29(20):2339
22. Nachemson, A., *back pain and causes, diagnosis and treatment updated in 1999*, S.C.o.T.A.i.H. care, Editor. 1999, Swedisch Council on Technology Assessment in Health Care. P.1-5.
23. OSHA, (Occupational safety and health administration), http://www.osha.gov/index.html, 15- 03 2009.
24. Poiraudeau S, Rannou F, Revel M, *Functional restoration programs for low back pain: a systematic review*, Annales de Réadaptation et de Medicine Physique, Volume 50, Issue 6, July 2007, Pages 425-429.
25. Sarno JE. Healing *Back Pain: The Mind-Body Connection.* Warner Books, 1991.

26. Shrey, D., & Hursh, N. (1999, 9). *Workplace Disability Management: International Trends and Perspectives*. Journal of Occupational Rehabilitation, pp. 45-52.
27. Simmons MJ, Kumar S. Lechelt E. "*Psychological factors in disabling low back pain: causes or consequences?*" Disability & Rehabilitation. 18(4): 161-8, 1996.
28. Stenger EM. "*Chronic back pain: view from a psychiatrist's office.*" Clinical Journal of Pain. 8(3): 242-6, 1992.
29. Van Oostrom SH, Anema JR, Terluin B, Venema A, de Vet HC, van Mechelen W. *Development of a workplace intervention for sick-listed employees with stress-related mental disorders: Intervention Mapping as a useful tool*. BMC Health Serv Res. 2007;7:127.
30. Waddell G. Volvo, *award in clinical sciences: a new clinical model for the treatment of low back pain*. Spine 1987;12:632–44.
31. Waddell G. *pain and disability*. The back pain revolution, 2nd edition, Churchill Livingstone, 2004: 27-45
32. Walker JM,. *Difference Between Disability and Impairment*: Journal of Occupational Rehabilitation, VoL 3, No. 3, 1993
33. Wheeler AH, Hanley EN Jr. *Nonoperative treatment for low back pain. Rest to restoration*, Spine 1995; 20(3): 375-378.
34. Whitaker, S. (2001). *The Management of sickness absence*. Occupational Environmental Medicine , pp. 420-424.
35. World Health Organization (WHO), http://www.who.int/en, 12-03 2009.

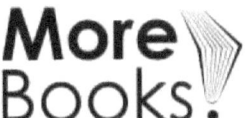
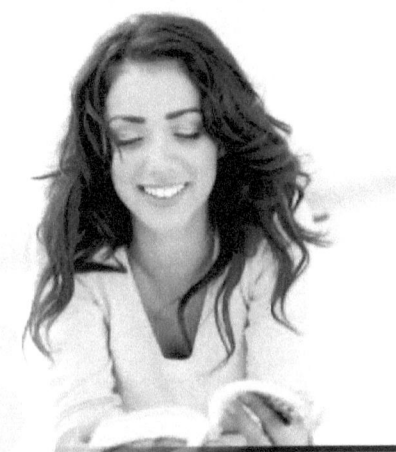

I want morebooks!

Buy your books fast and straightforward online - at one of world's fastest growing online book stores! Environmentally sound due to Print-on-Demand technologies.

Buy your books online at
www.morebooks.shop

Kaufen Sie Ihre Bücher schnell und unkompliziert online – auf einer der am schnellsten wachsenden Buchhandelsplattformen weltweit! Dank Print-On-Demand umwelt- und ressourcenschonend produziert.

Bücher schneller online kaufen
www.morebooks.shop

KS OmniScriptum Publishing
Brivibas gatve 197
LV-1039 Riga, Latvia
Telefax: +371 686 204 55

info@omniscriptum.com
www.omniscriptum.com

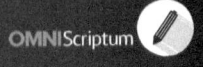

www.ingramcontent.com/pod-product-compliance
Lightning Source LLC
Chambersburg PA
CBHW031550210526
45464CB00003B/1243